Basic First Aid Management

A Book On First Aid And

Responding To Emergencies

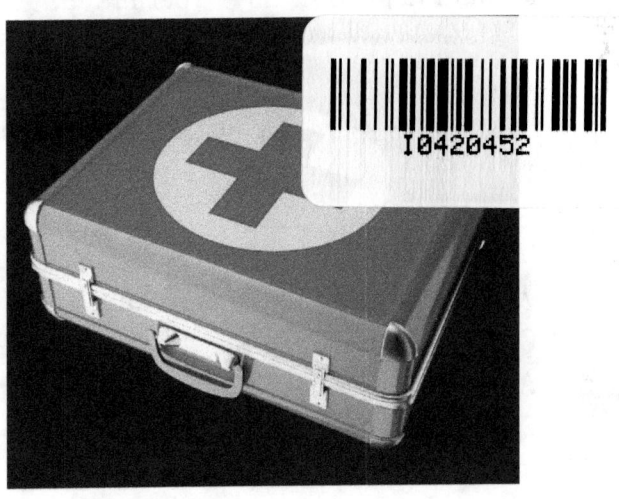

By

Paolo Jose de Luna

Paolo Jose de Luna

Copyright 2015 by Content Arcade Publishing - All rights reserved.

This document is geared towards providing exact and reliable information in regards to the topic and issue covered. The publication is sold with the idea that the publisher is not required to render accounting, officially permitted, or otherwise, qualified services. If advice is necessary, legal or professional, a practiced individual in the profession should be ordered.

- From a Declaration of Principles which was accepted and approved equally by a Committee of the American Bar Association and a Committee of Publishers and Associations.

In no way is it legal to reproduce, duplicate, or transmit any part of this document in either electronic means or in printed format. Recording of this publication is strictly prohibited and any storage of this document is not allowed unless with written permission from the publisher. All rights reserved.

The information provided herein is stated to be truthful and consistent, in that any liability, in terms of inattention or otherwise, by any usage or abuse of any policies, processes, or directions contained within is the solitary and utter responsibility of the recipient reader. Under no circumstances will any legal responsibility or blame be held against the publisher for any reparation, damages, or monetary loss due to the information herein, either directly or indirectly.

Respective authors own all copyrights not held by the publisher.

The information herein is offered for informational purposes solely, and is universal as so. The presentation of the information is without contract or any type of guarantee assurance.

Paolo Jose de Luna

The trademarks that are used are without any consent, and the publication of the trademark is without permission or backing by the trademark owner. All trademarks and brands within this book are for clarifying purposes only and are the owned by the owners themselves, not affiliated with this document.

Paolo Jose de Luna

Table of Contents

INTRODUCTION

No one can ever tell when an emergency hits. That's the thing about emergency situations, you can never tell when and where they'll happen, and whom they'll happen to. Oftentimes, emergencies result in the injury of one or more person, requiring immediate medical attention as it can lead to a number of complications or even death if not brought to the hospital immediately. But as an ordinary person without the background for medicine, how can you respond properly to these kinds of emergencies? Not too worry as we've got you all covered.

First aid is the solution that is given to that kind of problem. With first aid, one can respond to all sorts of emergencies and help treat injuries with utmost efficiency, speed, and resourcefulness. A common misconception made by a lot of people is that only those trained in healthcare like doctors and nurses are the only ones who can respond to emergencies and treat injuries – and that's dead wrong. First aid allows anyone, regardless of occupation, to respond to emergency situations and treat injuries of those involved in the incident. And most often, applying first aid can save the lives of many people.

First aid has a broad range of coverage. It covers treating cuts, bruises, burns, and sprains, up to responding to more serious problems like stroke, fractures, meningitis, and chemical emergencies. With the vast knowledge that you gain from first aid, you are able to help people that sustain injuries from various situations and you can save their lives in their time of need. Because of how first aid is more inclined to be considered as a medical practice, it actually teaches the basics when it comes to healthcare and responding to emergency situations because the goal of first aid isn't treatment but stabilization. At the end of each first aid, you'll notice how the final step would always be to call 911 or have someone call 911 or your local emergency response team. Through first aid, you allow the injured person to gain more time to get to the hospital where they can get adequate treatment in the emergency room with the use of medications, be tended by nurses, and be examined by doctors.

There are a number of institutions that provide first aid training, but you can also learn the basics of first aid by reading it from various resources online or in books. Practical training, however, is still the best way on learning first aid as it not only trains your knowledge in applying first aid, but you also gain the necessary skills when it comes to saving the lives of those who sustain injuries from emergency situations.

In this Book, you'll be able to learn the basics of first aid, how to respond to all sorts of emergencies, what to do when it comes to applying first aid for various types of situations ranging from simple fractures up to helping a person who had a heart attack. Gain the skills that are necessary for applying first aid and train yourself to develop the necessary skills to help those in need and save lives.

What is First Aid?

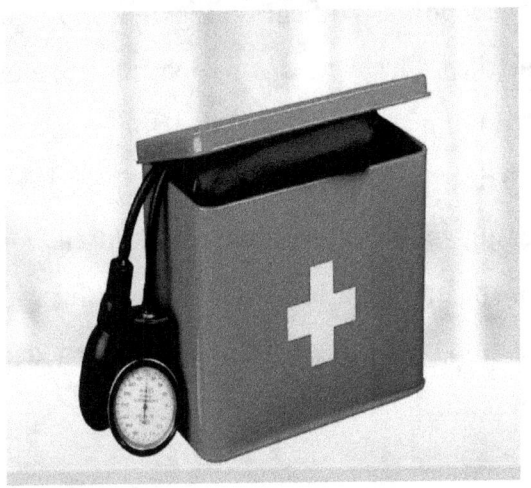

First aid, in its essence, is the application of emergency treatment to those who have sustained injuries or suffered from existing health problems. It is often known for its fast and efficient delivery of care, saving the lives of millions of people worldwide on a daily basis. Knowledge and skills on first aid is one of the basic requirements for those who want to work in the medical field and for those who want to work as emergency responders like police officers, firefighters, and medics. First aid can be learned through studying and training from several institutions worldwide, with Red Cross being one of the most well-known non-profit organizations that provide first aid training for those who are willing to learn first aid.

While first aid is considered to be the basic of the basics of applying healthcare treatment, it is considered as a foundation of everything else when it comes to stabilization of patients on various health conditions. But compared to the formal education that takes a number of years for healthcare professions, first aid can be learned in a matter of months or even days through teaching didactics and training necessary skills used in first aid.

Another thing that's unique about first aid is that it can be learned by anyone. You've got that right – it can be learned by *anyone*. May it be you're an engineer, a teacher, a teenager, an office worker, or a driver, you can learn first aid and you should learn first aid. It can save lives and learning first aid can help you and a lot of people.

There are a lot of places that you can learn first aid. Non-profit organizations like the Red Cross conduct frequent trainings for those who want to learn first aid. If you are one of the many people who want to learn first and help people during dire situations, then get your mind and body ready as you can gear up and train yourself in first aid by undergoing an easy procedure through registration and then participating in training. First aid training ranges from applying basic treatment for common injuries up to applying cardiopulmonary resuscitation or CPR. And with first aid, you are certain to save someone's life.

There are also advanced first aid courses that you can take, namely basic life support or BLS, advanced cardiac life support or ACLS, and pediatric advanced life support or PALS. These trainings are often undertaken by those in the medical profession or those who work in healthcare correlated professions. However, these courses can also be taken by anyone who want to learn the necessary skills to apply them in saving the lives of people.

In Basic Life Support (BLS), basic first aid training is included, but focuses more on saving people with the use of CPR. In Advanced Cardiac Life Support (ACLS), it involves a higher tier of BLS which involves learning CPR along with responding to a fast-paced emergency situation of a person having a heart attack and reading specific cardiac rhythms, applying corresponding treatments like administering shock or giving cardiac medication at the right time and at the right dose. In Pediatric Advanced Life Support (PALS), the focus lies more on applying emergency treatment for children and infants, saving their lives during cardiac emergencies and responding to accidents involving pediatric patients. Among these three advanced trainings, first aid still serves as the foundation stone for establishing the different disciplines and skills involved in saving the lives of people.

Today, first aid training is offered to those who want to be involved in treating people in emergency situations like for emergency medical team members, police officers, nurses, firefighters, and even students. There are no special requirements if you want to learn first aid, except for a medical certificate that proves you are in good health to participate in the training since first aid can be demanding both physically and mentally.

If you want to learn first aid, you can contact your local first aid training center or go to the nearest Red Cross center in your town. Most often, first aid training is offered for a small amount of fee, while the more advanced courses like BLS, ACLS, and PALS require a much higher fee because of its specialization.

Allergies and Anaphylaxis

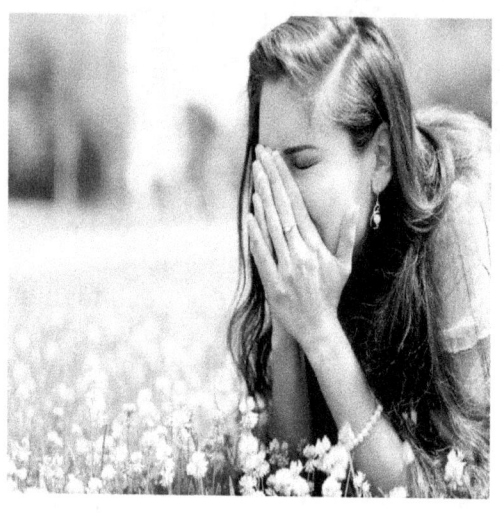

Allergies may develop from various sources such as pollen, dust, latex, certain types of food, and insect bites. Most often, rashes, itchiness or redness of the skin can develop, but more serious signs and symptoms can arise like swelling of the affected area, difficulty in breathing, diarrhea, nausea, vomiting, change in mental status, and shock. If left untreated, this can lead to a more severe case of allergic   reaction   called   *anaphylactic shock.*

In anaphylactic shock, breathing becomes much more difficult for the person and may lead to a decrease in blood pressure and thread pulse rate along with a decreased level of consciousness. If someone is at risk for developing an anaphylactic shock, they are usually prescribed with an Epi-pen® or epinephrine auto-injector to counteract the allergic reaction.

To give first aid treatment for those who are suffering from allergic reactions or anaphylaxis, here are the steps that you should follow:

- Once you identify a severe allergic reaction, immediately call 911 or your local EMTs number for help.

- Give them constant reassurance while waiting for the ambulance.

- If the person has an Epi-pen® available, here are the additional steps that you should follow in using it:

o Confirm that the Epi-pen® is prescribed for the person with allergy or anaphylactic shock.

o Before giving the shot, check the expiration date to confirm that the medication is still safe to use. If the medication inside the injector is visible, make sure that the liquid is clear. If the Epi-pen® is already expired or the liquid is cloudy, don't administer the medication.

o   Locate the middle outer portion of the person's thigh, making sure that there are no objects such as keys, mobile phones, or coins that obstruct the site. If you get consent, you can remove the pants or trousers of the person for a more effective way to administer the medication.

o   Grasp the Epi-pen® with the needle pointing down while your other hand pulls on the safety cap without bending or twisting it.

o   Hold the Epi-pen® perpendicularly to the injection site.

o   Push the tip of the Epi-pen® to the middle portion of the outer thigh.

o   Hold the Epi-pen® firmly in place for 10 seconds and administer the medication.

o   Remove the Epi-pen® from the thigh and massage the injection site or have the person massage the injection site for faster absorption of the medication.

○ Once you're done, check for the person's breathing to see if there are any improvements from the medication.

○ Reassure the person and try to keep them calm until help arrives.

○ If the EMTs are delayed and the person's allergic reaction does not respond to the medication, you can administer a second dose of the Epi-pen® using the same method above.

Be careful as different people respond to different items when it comes to stimulating their allergies. Some people may be allergic to certain food items like nuts, chicken, shrimp, crabs, or even dairy products. Always make sure that you ask a person for allergies if you are preparing food for them to avoid stimulating allergic reactions.

Some allergic reactions also come from insect bites particularly from bees and wasps. For those who display signs and symptoms of allergic reactions after being stung by a bee or a wasp, make sure you call 911 or your local EMTs immediately.

Paolo Jose de Luna

Asthma Attacks

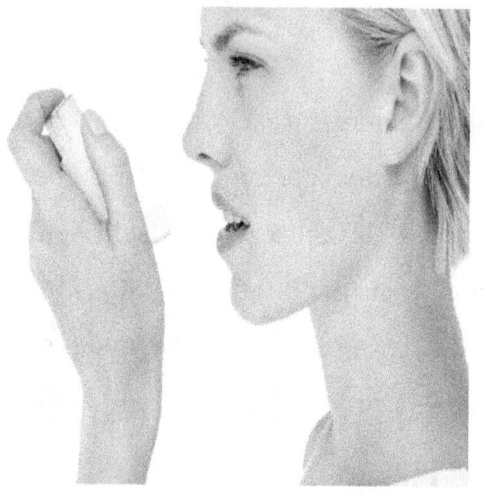

Asthma is one of the most common medical conditions in the world today, accounting for millions of hospitalizations each year. However, asthma, though it can be serious, can be managed at home with medications and therapies that help control the signs and symptoms. In asthma, the airways become narrowed and it makes it difficult to breathe in and out, resulting in additional distress on the part of the asthmatic person. Asthma can be diagnosed early in childhood and may eventually grow out of the person. However, asthma can still be present in adults, resulting in difficulty of breathing during episodes of anxiety, allergies, and stress.

You can tell if a person is having an asthma attack if they let you know. You also have to observe for difficulty of breathing, difficulty in speaking, coughing, and wheezing. A person having an asthma attack may feel distress, feel an impending sense of doom, and appear anxious as they have difficulty in breathing. In the most severe cases, asthma can result in the person having their lips, nail beds, and ears turn pale and then greyish to blue because of the lack of oxygen in their body.

Because asthma is one of the most common medical conditions in the world, applying first aid for the person having an asthma attack is essential to save their lives. Fortunately, it's easy to apply first aid to a person having an asthma attack.

Here are the steps that you should follow:

•   Help the person to sit in a comfortable position. When you're outdoors, you can have them sit in a shaded and comfortable area that is less crowded by people to allow them to breathe easier.

•   Help the person take their medication if they've brought their inhaler.

- You can also use a paper bag to let the person breathe in and out of to allow them to ease their breathing. This prevents the excessive blowing out of carbon dioxide from the lungs and eases the effort of the lungs during an asthma attack.

- Reassure the person and try to keep them calm.

- If the person having an asthma attack doesn't have their medication or if the signs and symptoms of asthma don't improve even after administering the medication, call 911 or your local EMTs for help.

Paolo Jose de Luna

Bleeding and Wounds

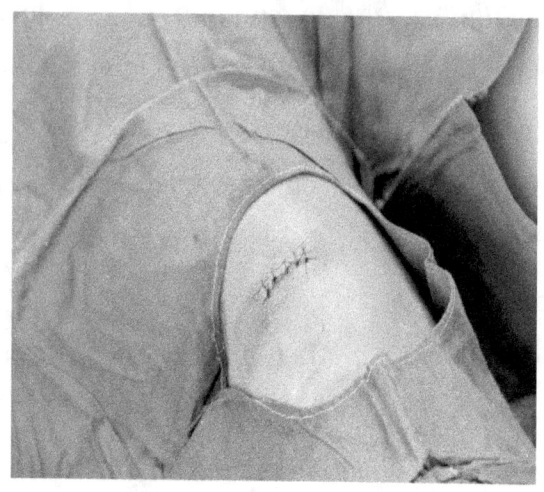

Injuries like cuts, abrasions, and gashes aren't anything new. These types of injuries can come from all sorts of incidents like accidents, falling over, hitting something hard, or attacks fueled violence. Regardless of the cause, administering first aid to these types of injuries is crucial because you can save the life of whomever received the injury.

While some may back away after seeing the sight of blood, it's actually isn't that difficult when it comes to giving first aid for bleeding and all sorts of wounds. Here are the steps that you should follow on how to give first aid for bleeding wounds:

- Apply pressure on the wound with whatever you can find. It doesn't have to be a sterile gauze coming from a first aid kit – it can be anything from your hand, a shirt, a towel, a cloth, or just about anything that can stop the bleeding and act as a plug to the wound. The pressure will allow the blood to clot and stop the bleeding.
- If the bleeding soaks the item that you have used, don't remove it from the wound but add more items like shirts and towels to maintain the pressure on the

area of bleeding and call 911 or your local EMTs as soon as possible. Extensive bleeding like this may indicate a major artery has been hit or cut.

- Raise the area where the bleeding is coming from, most often the arm or the leg, above the heart to minimize the bleeding further.

- For cases of nosebleeds, instruct the person to pinch their nose and lead forward. While leaning backwards may be the common thing to do, it isn't advised as it can only lead to the blood backing up into the airways and end up aspirating. Pinching the nose helps the blood to clot.

- Observe for any changes in consciousness, paleness, cold extremities, and dizziness as these are signs and symptoms of shock.

- If the bleeding is severe, call 911 or your local EMTs immediately.
- Keep putting pressure on the wound until help arrives.
- Continue to reassure the person and try to keep them calm until help arrives.

A common concern for people helping out in cases of bleeding is infection. While washing the wound is advised for smaller wounds and cuts, it isn't advised for wounds that bleed heavily. This is because the water will only wash away the clotting agents in the blood, interfering with the clotting and stopping the bleeding. As always, you should always institute standard precautions as you can never know what you can catch from someone else's blood. If you're unsure, always use gloves, a plastic bag, or have the person apply pressure on their wound themselves.

Paolo Jose de Luna

Burn Injuries

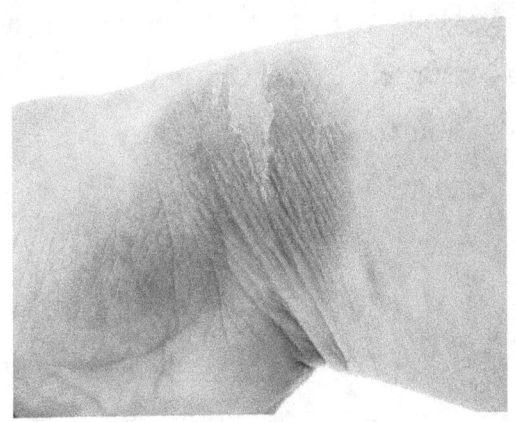

Just like cuts and abrasions, burns are also common injuries that can occur in the home. Burns usually occur from the kitchen, during cooking, serving a hot meal, fixing a stove, or handling hot liquids. Burns should be treated as serious injuries and here are the steps that you should take when it comes to administering first aid for burn injuries:

- Cool the burn by putting under cool running water for at least 10 minutes.

This will reduce the pain, redness, and swelling of the wound, as well as reducing the chances of scarring. The longer and the faster that the burn injury is cooled down, the less impact the injury has.

- If the burn needs medical management, cover the burn wound with a loose and clean dressing. This will prevent the area from infection since burn wounds are prone to develop infections.

- If the burn is serious (e.g. effects more than one area of the body, covers the hands, covers the joint, covers the face, develops blisters, underlying tissues can be seen, etc.) or if a child is burned, call 911 or your local EMTs immediately.

- Never put butter or toothpaste on the burn wound since these only worsen the burn. Though it's a common myth that these can help alleviate the pain of the burn, these will only retain the heat on the burn wound. Never put anything on the burn as these need to be removed later at the hospital, potentially causing further damage and pain.

• Never use ice to cool the burn as this may only worsen the burn injury. Use cool water for the burn. If you don't have any water available in the vicinity, use any other cold and running fluid.

• Never put adhesive bandages on the burn wound as they tend to stick hard to the burn, further causing injury. Loosely cover the burn with a dry and non-adhesive dressing to help prevent infection.

• If clothes are stuck to the burn, don't try to remove them as this may only cause further damage. Do remove the clothes and jewelries **around** the burn area to allow medical responders to have better visualization of the burn area later on.

Choking

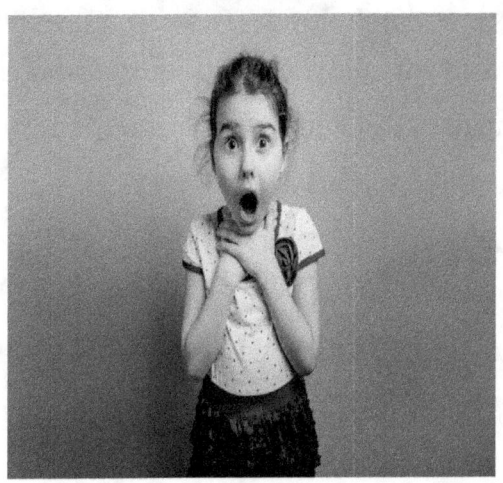

The respiratory system is an important organ system of the body, facilitating breathing through the lungs. Abnormality in the respiratory system brought about by the obstruction of the airways can result in severe complications or maybe even death if not treated immediately.

Obstruction of the airway, whether partial or complete, is considered as an immediate emergency. In first aid, you'll also be able to learn on how to give treatment and help out those who are choking. You need to act fast on your feet, identifying partial or complete airway obstruction when a person is choking as there are two ways to go about giving first aid to victims of choking. Here are the ways on how to give first aid for those who are choking:

• Go behind the person and hit firmly on the back between the shoulders up to five times to dislodge the object that may be obstructing the airway. Back blows are exceptionally useful for partial airway obstruction as there is still room for the object to get dislodged, set loose, and spit out by the choking person.

- If back blows don't remove the object obstructing the person's airway, give five quick abdominal thrusts. Stand behind the person, join your hands together and tie it around the victim's abdomen, forming a fist with your thumb sticking out perpendicularly to the victim's stomach.

- Pull your hands sharply and firmly with an inward and upward motion up to five times. This is also called the Heimlich maneuver and should never be attempted on a child under one year old as this can only cause more harm than good.

- Call 911 or your local EMTs when someone is choking.

- For a child, administering back blows and using the Heimlich maneuver can also be helpful when it comes to choking. However, never use the Heimlich maneuver on children under one year old. Don't hang the child by their feet as this can cause further dislodgement of the object that is obstructing their airway, making it more difficult to remove.

- For an infant that is choking, put their head lower than their chest, support their head and neck as you carry them on a prone position. Give five back blows between their shoulders and then five chest thrusts just below the nipple line. Repeat these steps until the object is forced out or if you can hear the baby cry.

Paolo Jose de Luna

Fractures, Strains and Sprains

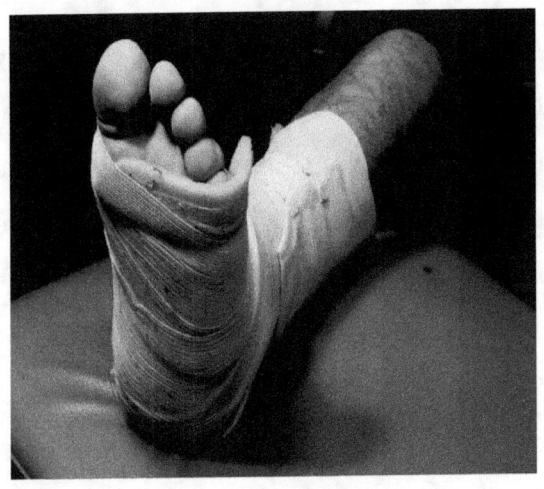

Among the many injuries incurred every day, fractures, strains, and sprains are common and can be treated at home if you know how to administer first aid properly. The musculoskeletal system is one of the most commonly injured body systems because of how it is used every day. Sports injuries are one of the usual causes of fractures, strains, and sprains, resulting in pain, discomfort, bruising, swelling, and redness of the affected area.

A fracture is a broken bone, usually brought about by an excessive amount of force that may have been placed upon the bone. A strain is when the muscle becomes overstretched through overuse and ends up getting damaged. A sprain is when a joint like the knee or wrist gets twisted and is damaged. For fractures, strains, and sprains, the first aid treatment is widely similar and should be learned by most.

Giving first aid for fractures and sprains require you to be calm, resourceful, and patient. It's one of the most basic principles learned in first aid and taking care of fractures, strains, and sprains isn't that challenging. Administering the RICE treatment is one of the most effective ways in handling fractures and sprains. Here are the steps that you should take when it comes to giving first aid to someone who has a fracture, strain, or sprain:

- Identify the area where the fracture or sprain has occurred to make sure what part of the body that you need to immobilize.
- Encourage the person to support the area of injury or use a cushion to prevent unnecessary movements of the fracture or sprain. This will minimize the pain and prevent further damage.
- **R**EST – Don't try to straighten out or move the injured area.

- **I**MMOBILIZE – Stabilize the injured area in the position that it was found. You can use a straight and hard object as a splint to prevent further movement of the injury. You can use things like rods, brooms, sticks, and anything that is straight and unmovable, tying it to the site of the injury.

- **C**OLD – Apply an ice pack to the injury to reduce the swelling, redness, and pain. If you don't have any ice available, you can use other things that are cold like frozen vegetables covered in a clean cloth. Leave the ice pack on the injury for about 20 minutes and remove it by then. Never apply ice directly on the injury as it can cause damage from ice burns.

- **E**LEVATE – Raise the injured part and the injured part only if it doesn't cause more pain and discomfort.

- Continue to reassure and keep the victim calm.
- Most of these injuries respond to the application of a cold compress. If the injury doesn't respond to the first aid treatment or if you suspect a broken bone, call 911 or your local EMTs immediately for further management.
- Never use a warm towel or alternate between warm and cold compresses. The most effective way to reduce pain and swelling in bone and muscle injuries is by applying a cold compress.

Among the many first aid principles, administering first aid to fractures, strains, and sprains is one of the most common. It will do you well if you learn on how to apply first aid to a broken bone, a damaged joint, or an overstretched muscle because of how frequent it can occur at home, in school, at work, or even out in the streets.

Unconsciousness

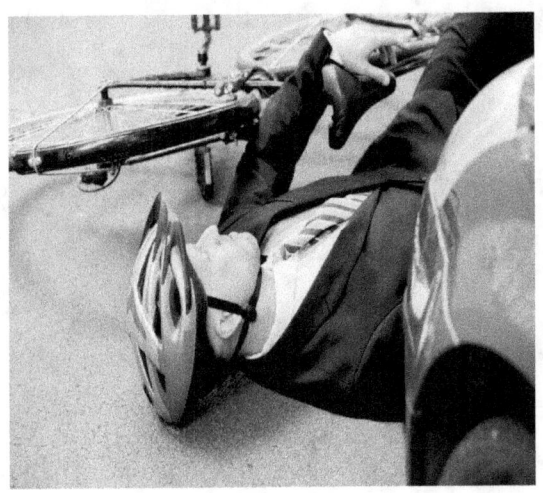

Seeing someone faint and then fall unconscious can be a distressing experience, even for the experienced healthcare provider. Most often, unconsciousness may indicate an underlying health condition that should be treated immediately. The role of first aid here is to stabilize the patient and ensure that they are in the optimum condition. When you see an unconscious individual, you should always check for their breathing and pulse as the first step to administering first aid. Here are the steps that you should follow in administering first aid treatment to someone who is unconscious:

• Check for breathing by tilting their head backwards, looking at the rise of their chest and feeling for their breaths. When a person falls unconscious, the muscles tend to relax and the tongue may block the airway, preventing the person from breathing normally. When you tilt their head, the airway is opened and the tongue is pulled backwards to open the airway. Look for the rise and fall of the chest while feeling for the victim's breaths on your cheeks.

- Call 911 or your local EMTs immediately or have someone else do it.

- If you can't feel for any breaths, proceed to check for pulse by sliding your three fingers on the victim's neck, palpating their carotid artery. The carotids can easily be felt compared to the radial pulse since the artery is bigger and you only need to do this for a second.

- If you've confirmed that there are no breaths and the pulses are absent, immediately start doing cardiopulmonary resuscitation or CPR.

- Place the heel of your hand on the center of the victim's chest while the heel of the other hand is placed on top of the first hand, intertwining your fingers together.

- Start delivering chest compressions by firmly pushing downwards in the middle of the chest about 2 inches deep and then release. Push hard and push fast, making sure that your elbows are kept locked and straight.

- Chest compressions make sure that blood is pumped throughout the body and helps the vital organs, including the brain, alive by mimicking the pumping action of the heart and it can even dislodge anything that may obstruct the airway.

- Keep delivering chest compressions at a rate of 100 chest compressions per minutes.

- Give 2 rescue breaths for every 30 chest compressions:

o   Tilt the head backwards and lift the chin upwards.

o   Pinch the nose to create a complete seal over the victim's mouth.

o   Blow in for about a second and watch for the chest rise.

o   Give 2 rescue breaths, one after the other.

o   If the chest does not rise with the rescue breaths, tilt the head of the victim again and give another rescue breath.

• Continue giving CPR until help arrives or if these situations arise:

o   You observe an obvious sign of life (e.g. breathing, waking up, etc.)

o   An Automatic External Defibrillator or AED is available and ready to use.

o   Another trained responder or an EMT is now on the scene.

o   You are too tired to continue giving CPR.

o   The scene becomes unsafe for you and the victim.

- Once you see obvious signs of life, you can stop doing CPR.

- Place the victim on to their side. This will prevent them from aspirating from their own saliva that may have accumulated during the period of unconsciousness. This is called the recovery position.

- Tilt their head backwards. If you suspect a neck or back injury, it is still advised to tilt the victim's head backwards since your priority here is to promote breathing. Ensure that their spine is kept in a straight line. If you don't know what to do, ask someone for help, call 911 or your local EMTs immediately.

- If you find someone unconscious and not breathing, call for help before you start giving chest compressions. This way, you can save time and administer chest compressions while making sure that help is on the way.

- If there is someone with you, alternate doing chest compressions for about one to two minutes with minimal interruptions in between, until help arrives. Don't worry about injuring the ribs of the victim as the ribs can heal in time. Without CPR, the chances of survival for the victim will be low.

- Once the person shows signs of life and you've put them on their side, keep monitoring the victim's breathing, pulse, and level of consciousness until help arrives.

CONCLUSION

Responding to an emergency situation can be a challenge at first, especially if you are inexperienced. The most important thing that you should remember is that you should keep your cool and keep yourself from panicking. Most often, a lot of people fail to administer competent first aid treatment because of their worry, anxiety, and panicking over the victim. When it comes to first aid, keeping calm should always be the first step that you should take and keeping a clear mind will allow you to make the best decisions for any given situation. Don't be afraid and be confident when it comes to administering first aid.

First aid allows you to administer emergency medical treatment for various situations. May it be bleeding, allergies, or heart attacks, the priority of first aid is to administer fast and immediate treatment to increase the victim's survival rate until help arrives or until they get to the hospital. The goal of first aid isn't to provide a complete cure for the victim, but rather to provide emergency treatment and to stabilize the victim's condition. You'll notice this as there is always calling 911 or the local EMTs as a step to every medical emergency you've read so far in this Book. Always remember these goals whenever you administer first aid treatment.

First aid covers more topics that you should read about. This eBook features the most common emergencies that you may respond to in the future. Hopefully, this eBook has helped you shed light upon the different medical emergencies that may arise in different places, may it be at home, in school, at work, or even around your neighborhood.

Be ready and be prepared – that's what first aid is all about.